Aromatherapy Basics

Other Books by Penny Keay

Aromatherapy Recipes using Pure Essential oils Volume 1

Breads from the Heart

Aromatherapy Basics

Penny & Alan Keay

Penny Keay

Penny Makes Cents, LLC

Minnesota, USA

First Published in the United States in 2013

ISBN 978-0-9822142-6-8

Printed in the U.S.A.

Dedication:

Those interested in learning all about the use of essential oils as used in aromatherapy for your health and well-being.

Table of Contents

Cover Photo © Penny Keay

Graphics and Photography throughout this book are licensed for use by 123rf.com

PREFACE

This book is a basic guide for anyone interested in the proper and safe use of essential oils as used in therapeutic aromatherapy. It will give you the 'basics'.

Of course, it will also provide you with general helps for those that just want to enjoy essential oils throughout their daily lives.

Getting started in Aromatherapy can be very overwhelming.

The information presented is the 'beginning' and basic information everyone should read before purchasing that first bottle of essential oil.

We are providing you with information to help you learn in baby steps. Over the years, we have heard it very often that aromatherapy seems almost too much to comprehend.

This book is not a 'history' of aromatherapy, nor is it a 'chemistry' of aromatherapy. Those areas are some things that can overwhelm you when you are first introduced to aromatherapy.

They are not needed at the beginning. They will only be needed if you decide to become very serious to pursue further education and certifications.

This is a book to help you get 'started', to help you understand what essential oils are, where good oils come from, how to buy and how to use them safely and responsibly.

It will briefly introduce you on how to use them for yourself and others for your health and well-being. We try to give you answers to some of the things you will encounter as you start your Aromatherapy journey.

As we stated with the title of the book, this is a Basic Aromatherapy book to introduce you to the use of essential oils.

Once you understand the information presented you will feel more confident when you are seeking essential oils for your own personal use or when sharing them with others in your life.

Without further ado, Let the Journey begin!

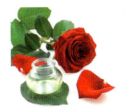

WHAT IS AROMATHERAPY?

Aromatherapy means simply - the study of scents used in a therapeutic manner, usually by inhalation or diffusing into the air.

The more detailed definition is the skilled and controlled use of essential oils for emotional and physical health and well-being.

The practice of aromatherapy goes beyond smell, though.

It involves "pure" essential oils and treatments that many believe may have a chemical effect on the body.

Apply essential oils by massage, put in the bath, diffused in the air, added to hair and skin care products and many other applications.

Aromatherapy is a system of enabling the body to help heal itself by providing basic chemical constituents of the plants that the body may be missing or possibly out of balance.

In Europe and other parts of the world, but not so much in the USA, medical doctors prescribe essential oils, for internal use.

According to the limitations set by the Food and Drug Administration pure undiluted essential oils in the USA cannot be ingested unless prescribed by a licensed medical professional. Otherwise, they need to be diluted according to the USDA regulations for use as a food flavoring ingredient.

Lately there are companies claiming their products are "Aromatherapy such and such". They advertise things such as candles and various bath products. Although these products may smell nice, they are not necessarily therapeutic.

PLEASE be aware that this is not the THERAPEUTIC AROMATHERAPY as we practice.

What they are advertising are "scents" that undoubtedly will make you feel good, but they are not necessarily made with 100% Pure Essential oils but the scents may be made with artificially, made petroleum based fragrances.

Fragrance oils do not always contain the pure plant essence that has the true, natural, healing properties.

Alternative or Complementary

Although listed as an Alternative Health modality, most aroma therapists prefer to call it Complementary Health care.

Do not use Aromatherapy to replace your regular health care, but as an addition to compliment your health care program and support your well-being.

Please be sure to keep your Health Care Provider informed when you choose to use Essential oils and Aromatherapy as part of your health care regimen.

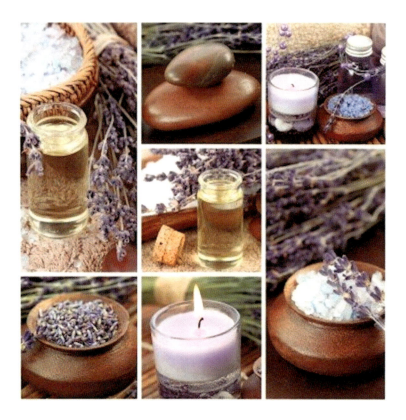

The Different Types of Aromatherapy

There are several ways to implement aromatherapy.

The practice of Holistic Therapeutic Aromatherapy is one such type and is the main scope of this book. Holistic Aromatherapy involves looking at the body as a whole.

This means choosing the right essential oils to bring about the intended results for the physical and emotional well-being of the persons seeking help. As a holistic aroma therapist, we may look at diet, environmental factors such as home or working conditions. We look at the whole not just a part of a person's given situation.

Other types of Aromatherapy are practiced by Massage Therapists, Nursing Staff and Medical doctors, Esthetics, Psychological, Spiritual leaders (essential oils are used throughout the world in religious and other ritual ceremonies) and for use with Animals.

Nevertheless, no matter what category of aromatherapy they all use essential oils in the practice. Moreover, many of these types are interlinked.

WHAT ARE ESSENTIAL OILS?

Essential oils are the subtle, volatile liquids distilled from plants, shrubs, flowers, trees, bushes and seeds. Pressing the peels from citrus fruits will also produce essential oils.

An ancient process, oil distillation is a delicate and precise art until recently was almost forgotten.

Science is just now re-discovering the incredible healing power of essential oils.

Essential oils oftentimes regarded as the 'life blood' of the plant kingdom.

Science and medicine are now beginning to acknowledge their value in physical and mental health care.

Essential oils are known for their immune stimulating, anti-viral, anti-infectious, anti-bacterial, antimicrobial, anti-septic, anti-tumoral, anti-fungal, and anti-parasitic properties.

They can be Stimulating, Uplifting, Relaxing, Calming. They can help with Memory, Focusing and Mental alertness.

Many folks use them while at work, at school, before and after sports, while meditating and much more.

There is a long list of health concerns essential oils can be helpful when used properly.

HISTORY OF AROMATHERAPY

The history of aromatherapy goes back thousands of years. Although not called Aromatherapy until the early 1900's. Aromatic plants and essential oils were often used in biblical times. (Think of the gifts brought to the new born.)

Plant oils are mentioned several times in the Bible. In addition, Cleopatra used essential oils in her perfumery.

Ancient Greeks and Romans used the oils in their medical treatments. The Egyptians used aromatic plant essences to treat both physical and mental health problems. In the East, China and India, doctors also knew the therapeutic benefits of plant essences.
Today's Aromatherapy and concepts began with a French chemist, René-Maurice Gattefossé. He coined the term "aromatherapie".

He was convinced that the oils had antiseptic properties - more powerful than the antiseptics used at that time (1920's). He also knew that they had other important healing abilities.

While conducting an experiment in distillation he burned his hand and needing to cool it down, put his entire hand into a vat of pure lavender essential oil.

The pain was gone almost instantly. Over the next few days, his burn healed with no blisters, scars or infections. Thereafter he continued his research of this incredible phenomenon and uses of essential oils for other possible medical uses.

In Europe and other parts of the world, medical practitioners prescribe essential oils for internal use, massages etc.

In the USA, Aromatherapy is part of the cosmetics industry and regulated by the FDA when used for scenting and perfumery. On the other hand, if they are used in foods and flavoring they are regulated by the USDA.

PARTS OF THE PLANTS THAT ARE USED

The part of the plant that is used often times will correlate to the part of the human body where it is used or is most beneficial.

Of course, essential oils will affect the whole body to varying degrees depending on the expected applications purpose.

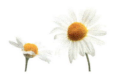 **Flowers/Blossoms** affect the nervous and endocrine systems, which means, these oils have a calming, relaxing, intoxicating, aphrodisiac and spiritual reaction.

Some of those oils are rose, jasmine, neroli, ylang ylang, chamomiles, lavender and clary sage.

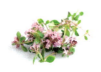 **Flowers/Plants** affect the nervous and endocrine systems with a stimulating, energizing, refreshing affect.

Some of those oils are basil, peppermint, spearmint, rosemary, lavender and (pictured) thyme.

Leaves affect the respiratory system to help with breathing, opening and cleansing of the system.

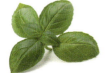 Some of those oils are basil (pictured), eucalyptus, geranium, myrtle, petitgrain and tea tree.

Also included in this list are the needle oils, which are the firs, pine and spruce.

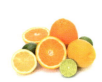 **Fruit/Peel/Rinds** affect the cardiovascular (heart and blood) and the lymphatic (elimination) systems to help with well-being, warming and uplifting.

Some of those oils are bergamot, orange, lemon, mandarin and grapefruit.

 Fruit/Seeds affect the digestive and lymphatic systems with balancing and revitalizing.

Some of those oils are caraway, carrot, clove bud (pictured) cumin and black pepper.

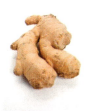

Roots affect the intestinal system to help with grounding and connecting to Mother Earth.

Some of those oils are angelica root vetiver, ginger (pictured) and valerian.

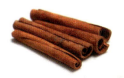

Wood/Resins affect the endocrine system with energy, inner strength, balancing.

Some of those wood oils are camphor, cedar, rosewood and sandalwood.

Some of those resin oils are; elemi, frankincense, myrrh and for bark the oil is cinnamon (pictured).

There are approximately 450 essential oils produced around the world for use in any variety of applications.

Essential oils mainly used in industry for food, flavoring, perfumery, but are also used for manufacturing many other products.

Only about 150 essential oils are used in Therapeutic Aromatherapy. In addition, of those 150, approximately 50 are those that will be useful for 95% of the applications necessary for the majority of health concerns.

For beginners starting out using essential oils, only about 10-12 are necessary to accommodate the everyday needs of most families.

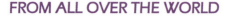

FROM ALL OVER THE WORLD

Essential oils come from all over the world.

Just to name a few, where they most commonly come from:

Sweet Orange from the USA, Ylang ylang from Madagascar and Comoros, Rose from Bulgaria and Turkey, Lavender from Bulgaria and France, Tea Tree from Australia, Sandalwood from India, Peppermint from the USA and several other countries.

The plants are grown in all kinds of climates and in a variety of geographic areas. These are important factors in the quality of essential oil produced in any given year.

Just like fine wines, each year's harvest can vary from year to year. In some years, superior oils are produced in abundance, whereas in subsequent years the oil produced may be minimal and poor quality or vice versa.

Controlled organic farming means the plants are grown in a no fertilizers, no pesticides or artificial herbicides environment.

Please note that many third world countries are where the plants are grown for essential oil production. They will not pay for herbicides or pesticides to produce essential oils, nor can they pay for to be certified organic.

The best way to know if essential oils are contaminant free is to have them tested by gas chromatography and mass spectrometry. Many other tests can be performed to assess purity.

Do not rely on the term 'organic' to mean the essential oil is therapeutic. The majority of essential oils will never be produced on 'organic' soils or under 'organic' conditions. In addition, even though they are not grown in organic soils, the essential oils produced may still be giving wonderful therapeutic results.

You are better off paying for oils that have undergone the above-mentioned testing, to assure you they are free from herbicides and pesticides. Meaning, the essential oils have the constituents as suggested by aroma therapeutic use.

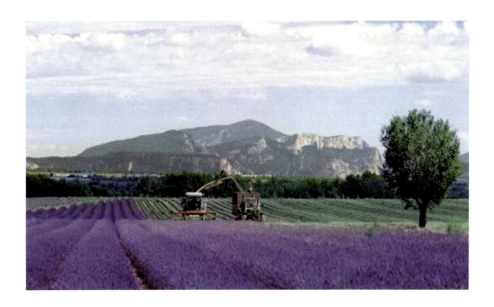

Lavender Flower Harvest in France

GET GOOD QUALITY

The aromas not only change from one part of the plant to another, they may also change due to weather, time of day and location at the time of harvesting and type of extraction methods used.

The quality, price and the strength of the essential oils vary according to variety or family of the plant, part of the plant used, and again the time of harvest (early morning or late afternoon), the method of distillation used and the type of soil grown in.

For therapeutic uses, try to get only oils that are pure and grown with no herbicides or pesticides.

Therapeutic oils are usually used by the drops, not by ounces or other measurements.

The one other thing that comes to mind when using 100% pure essential oils is what some people have said - "I'm allergic to lavender**(for example). I can't use that."

What most people do not realize is that they are not allergic to lavender BUT they are allergic to one or more of the chemicals used in making perfumed or synthetic oils.

Allergic reactions could be caused from the pollen produced by flowering plants.

There is no pollen in essential oils.

** People can be sensitive to any essential oil but true allergic reactions are rare.

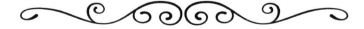

DO ESSENTIAL OILS HAVE A GRADE OR QUALITY RATING?

You might wonder about "Quality" or "Grade" of oils.

To help you have a better understanding of the quality of essential oils used in Therapeutic Aromatherapy, one thing you will need to understand is there is no 'grading' system established for essential oils in the USA or throughout the world. There are many, many essential oil suppliers throughout the world but not all essential oils are used in Therapeutic Aromatherapy.

In fact, the majority of essential oils are used in the food and flavoring industry. The next largest industry is the perfume industry.

Although essential oils are used in both of those industries and could possibly produce a therapeutic response, their quality is not dependent on providing the results sought after for massage or medical applications, or complementary medicine.

In the food, flavoring and perfumery industries, the flavor and especially the smell are of utmost importance.

If the essential oil(s) used in a particular formulation do not meet the expectation or requirement for that manufacturer, they will have their chemists 'manipulate' the oil with man-made chemicals to 'standardize' the 'end' product.

They want their finished product to always smell and or taste the same. They may start with the basic essential oil but most often, they will have been altered or what we call 'adulterated' to meet certain criteria specifically required by the food processor, manufacturer or perfumer.

Fragrance oils are usually made from a majority of fabricated laboratory created scents. They may have a few essential oils but the main components of fragrance oils are fabricated in a laboratory and have no therapeutic value.

Fragrance oils are often times detrimental to your health. They do not have a plant name nor do they have a botanical name. They have names like Fresh linens, Berries and Cream etc.

When trying to find essential oils that have not been manipulated by either the original farmer, during distillation or someone along the distribution chain, can be a challenge for anyone in the aromatherapy business.

When used in Therapeutic Aromatherapy, you want essential oils that have not been manipulated, and not standardized by a laboratory or been adulterated or diluted by anyone along the way.

The essential oils should be analyzed by laboratories that **specialize in therapeutic aromatherapy**. They know and understand the plants chemical makeup and what constituents are necessary and the percentages of those needed to provide the 'therapeutic' aromatherapy industry the essential oils that will produce medical and therapeutic result.

Grading - Grades of oils – plain and simple there is no such thing.

We must address this issue, as you will, without a doubt, run into somebody selling you the 'grading' of essential oils.

Well, to put it simply, there is no industry standard for 'Grading' essential oils.

No country around the world has a grading system in place for essential oils, not one.

Any company making claims their oils are 'graded therapeutic' are stretching the truth. You must understand that the 'grading' system 'they' use is strictly an 'in house' or that particular companies set of standards for adopting a 'grading' system for the essential oils they sell.

There are companies who may state their oils are "Therapeutic Grade" or Grade A or #1. Realize this just is not so. It is just THEIR system.

To reiterate - There is no industry grading system for essential oils. When you see this, you need to realize it is only 'their' system of grading essential oils.

It really does not tell you if they are pure, unadulterated essential oils. Namely, because we do not know what they are 'grading' their essential oils against for comparison.

Because in the Essential oil industry there are no set standards, there is no grading system.

Nevertheless, we can tell you this – there are different qualities of essential oils.

There are the pure unadulterated, as nature intended it to be, quality that is used by Therapeutic Aromatherapists.

There are the Perfumer quality oils that are manipulated to smell exactly the same from year to year.

There are the Food and Flavoring industry quality that again has been manipulated to not only smell the same but also taste the same as required by their customers.

In Summary about Quality:

Essential oils used in **therapeutic aromatherapy**

- Come from one plant species.

- Are not adulterated or 'standardized'

- Are processed and analyzed by Gas Spectrometry and Mass Chromatography to determine the chemical constituents and to identify any chemicals that should not be there. Several other tests may also be performed.

- Include their **Common name** and **Botanical (Latin) name** on their labels. Good labels should show the Country of origin and method of extraction.

- Prices will never be the same for all products being sold in a certain size bottle. 10 mL bottle of Rose oil, for example, is a hundred times more expensive than Orange oil.

- Are typically sold by people that take aromatherapy very seriously, these people are serious enough to get further education belong to professional organizations and know and follow safety guidelines for proper usage.

Essential oils used in Perfumery or the Food and Flavoring Industry or fragrance oils:

- Are often times manipulated to smell or taste a specific way and may be very 'cheap' with all scents priced the same for a particularly quantity.

- May not produce therapeutic results due to adulterations, additives may cause skin or other unpleasant reactions

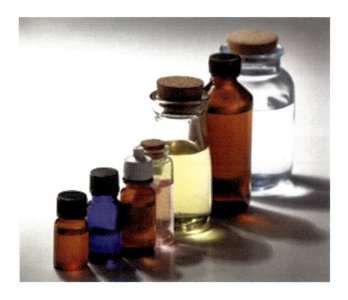

HOW ESSENTIAL OILS ARE EXTRACTED

There are a few different ways for the oils to be extracted.

Steam distillation is the most common way of extraction.

In this method, steam from boiling water is used to extract the oils from the plants. The steam is then cooled and condensed into a liquid where the oils are skimmed off as it floats on top of the water.

This produces a fairly high and good quality of oil.

Cold pressing is used to extract the oils by shredding, squeezing or pressing the oils out of the peel of the fruit without the use of heat. It really is not 'cold' as anytime you have any type of pressure there is some heat created but at a lower heat or temperature than when steam is created.

Solvent extraction - this method is more costly than the other types of extraction. It is more efficient and produces more oil especially from those plants and flowers that offer only extremely small quantities of essential oils or absolute.

Absolute flower oils and several vegetable oils are extracted by this method.

An absolute is the name given to essential oils extracted by solvent and CO_2 extraction.

It is possible that a toxic residue can remain with the solvent method of extraction. The oil, which it produces, may be non-pure oil.

Although in today's markets, the essential oils are often times further refined to produce a superior product safe to use.

Carbon dioxide or CO_2 - the oils are extracted under high pressure in a few minutes without chemical reaction or solvent residues.

This process is becoming more popular even though it is more expensive to do.

There are several other methods of extraction of essential oils and absolutes but they are usually not cost effective nor do they produce a usable quantity of oil.

DISTILLING ON YOUR OWN

For those wishing to distill their own essential oils - did you know that it takes 2,000 pounds of Rose petals to make a pound of Rose oil.

How about Eucalyptus - 50 pounds, or Lavender - 150 pounds, Rosemary takes 500 pounds and Jasmine - 1000 pounds of raw materials?

Of course, you do not need to distill such large quantities.

There is smaller scale distilling equipment available to fit your needs.

Realize though that even the smaller quantities will still take many pounds of plant material to produce a few milliliters of pure essential oils.

In addition, the equipment can be quite costly. We suggest that unless you plan on large-scale production, just purchase the essential oils you need!

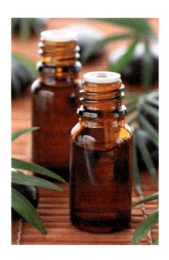

HOW OUR SENSE OF SMELL WORKS

With our sense of smell, we are able to identify up to 10,000 different smells!!

Some make us feel better while others make us shy away like bad odors or a bad memory.

Here is what happens when you smell something. The aroma enters the nasal cavity (and mouth to a small degree) and goes up to the olfactory nerves in our nostrils. Here the nerves react to the aroma and a signal is sent to the limbic system of the brain.

The limbic part of the brain is where motivation, emotion and certain kinds of memory are triggered.

It is here where all the aromas are "recognized" immediately, whereas the senses of taste, sound and touch are not as instantaneous.

Once the limbic brain is stimulated, it sends signals to the hypothalamus. The hypothalamus then involves the body and affects the mood, memory and neuroendocrine regulatory systems.

The brain has also a "lock and key" mechanism. This means that an aroma (the key) will give you the "memory" which has been 'locked' away since you first smelled it. So, whether it is good (like Grandma's freshly baked bread) or bad (like the "aroma" of a skunk!), it will trigger a memory.

Some aromas will tell the limbic system to release different chemicals. Such as endorphins, to help kill pain or induce sexual feelings, Serotonins to help relax or calm, Enkephalin's - help to reduce pain and give you a good feeling about yourself.

Aromas do help you feel better which makes the stress part of our lives a little easier to handle.

What happens if you have lost your sense of smell? Do not worry, since the sense of smell is not critical to the therapeutic effect of essential oils.

It is the chemical reactions the essential oils produce, starting within the nasal passage, continuing throughout the body that will produce the final outcome.

Many people will still benefit from the use of essential oils even if they cannot smell or taste anything.

In several cases throughout history, it is not unheard of for someone who had a diminished sense of smell, have it came back and with more acuity.

Aroma therapists will often times develop a keen sense of smell and due to the increased ability to smell, various odors will detest the artificial scents and fragrances used in many personal care and household cleaning products.

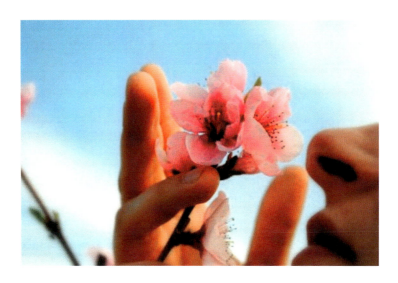

THE NOTES

The notes of essential oils and absolutes are a method to identify the scents, as they are smelled. The 'scale' was developed by a French perfumer Charles Piesse during the 19th century.

In actuality, it is also a method used to help to describe the evaporation rates of essential oils.

The notes are Top, Middle and Base

Top notes evaporate rather quickly, Middle notes are the heart and soul of a blend and the Base notes hold on and linger, grounding the blend.

Some essential oils will have components that will fit in to each 'note' category. Each note of that essential oil is excitingly different.

In a blend of essential oils, the first 'note' that is smelled is considered the Top note. Each essential oil will fit into one of the 'note' categories. The Top note is also called a 'head' note. Since these are the ones you will smell first!

Here are the ways to tell the difference in the notes (evaporation rate) of the oils.

Top notes:

- Evaporate in less than 2 hours
- Are the first aromas you smell
- Are stimulating and uplifting

Examples are basil, eucalyptus, lemon, lime, orange, peppermint, tea tree.

Middle notes:

- Take up to 4 hours to evaporate
- Make blends stay together better

Examples are chamomile, fennel, geranium, juniper, lavender, marjoram. melissa, black pepper.

Base notes:

- Take up to 6 hours or more to evaporate
- Helps hold blends together
- Are relaxing or 'grounding' oils

Examples are cedarwood, frankincense, jasmine, myrrh, patchouli, ylang ylang.

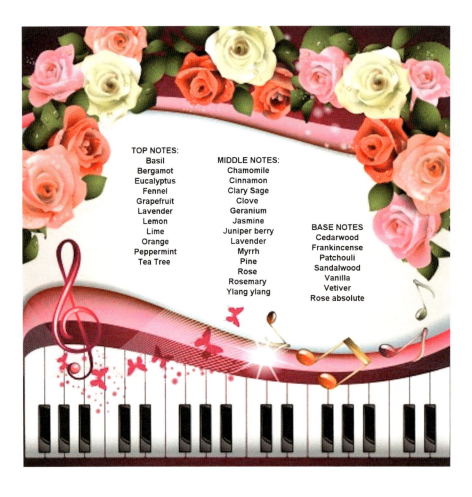

TOP NOTES:
Basil
Bergamot
Eucalyptus
Fennel
Grapefruit
Lavender
Lemon
Lime
Orange
Peppermint
Tea Tree

MIDDLE NOTES:
Chamomile
Cinnamon
Clary Sage
Clove
Geranium
Jasmine
Juniper berry
Lavender
Myrrh
Pine
Rose
Rosemary
Ylang ylang

BASE NOTES
Cedarwood
Frankincense
Patchouli
Sandalwood
Vanilla
Vetiver
Rose absolute

CARE OF ESSENTIAL OILS

Essential oils require a little extra care.

You should store your oils in glass bottles away from heat and light. Storing them in a cool place will prolong their quality.

The biggest destruction factor for essential oils is oxygen. Air will quickly oxidize, alter and destroy your precious essential oils.

The essential oils evaporate easily and should be stored in an air-tight bottle.

Do not allow a lot of 'empty' space in your bottle of oil. You should move the essential oils to a smaller bottle to prevent unnecessary oxidation.

Pure essential oils will evaporate without a trace, except those with high levels of pigmentation such as Yarrow and German Chamomile. Even Sweet or Blood Orange can stain clothing due to pigments they may leave behind.

Use all oils with respect. Learn their properties and know their actions.

ESSENTIAL OIL SAFETY

This is a very important aspect of aromatherapy. Essential oils are very potent and highly concentrated chemicals extracted from plants by distillation.

One needs to remember that only a drop or two of essential oils are needed in most applications. Most essential oils are safe to use but please use extra precautions around children, the elderly and pets.

An essential oil that can be used on one person or animal may not be suitable for another.

Use potentially toxic oils only as directed by a certified Aromatherapist or in dilutions as recommended in a recipe

Exception is cats – do not use essential oils around them at all. Their liver cannot metabolize the oils and the essential oils will ultimately cause liver failure or death.

If an essential oil is applied to the skin and starts an adverse reaction - clean the area with a fixed or carrier oil, such as almond, sesame etc, followed by soap and warm water.

If accidentally splashed into the eyes use full fat milk (not skim) to rinse, followed by a lot of clear water.

Water alone may not wash oil from eye(s) but the milk has fat in it that will help absorb the oil. Seek medical attention should you get a large amount splashed in your eyes.

Some essential oils are milder (Lavender) while others are extremely strong (Peppermint, Thyme and Oregano) when applied to the skin and when inhaled. Nevertheless, just because an essential oil may have a light smell does not mean it will not have strong properties for emotional and health reasons.

Any essential oil can be a potential poison, so caution needs to be used around children, pets and the elderly. When using recipes for children and the elderly, cut the essential oil amounts in half but always use the normal amount of carrier oils in massage, lotion or other applications. Then when applied, use only small amounts on children and the elderly.

Please keep all essential oils out of the reach of children! We do not mean just toddlers. Unless your teenager has been properly instructed, they too, should be using essential oils with adult supervision.

Some other major concerns are sensitization and skin irritations. A simple way to check to see if you have sensitive skin to any oil, you can test a small amount of essential oil (a drop diluted with carrier oil) on the inner arm (near the elbow). Observe for 24 hours, if no reaction, then you can proceed using on a routine basis. Of course, if at any time while using essential oils you see or feel an unpleasant reaction, discontinue use.

Any cold pressed or expressed citrus oil can cause a photosensitivity reaction to occur. If applied to the skin and then exposed to sunlight or UV light such as in tanning salons, discoloration and burn can occur. Avoid using citrus essential oils or blends for several hours prior to exposure to either of these.

Alternatively, you can use essential oils that have been stream distilled. In the case of Bergamot, use Bergamot FCF (Furo-coumarin Free) as this extraction of Bergamot is safe to use on skin should it be exposed to sunlight or UV rays.

What about using essential oils during pregnancy? Since most essential oils are found in everyday products like toothpaste, foods, and in household products many of them are also safe to use when pregnant.

Although to be on the safe side, using essential oils for other applications and just like any other drug or strong chemical, it is suggested, that most essential oils be avoided during the first trimester.

After those first three months, many essential oils can be used in moderation. Inhalation is preferred over skin applications. Again, when used in massage blends, follow the recommended recipe.

If the recipe pertains specifically to pregnancy you can follow the recipe as written or if the recipe is for the general population, cut the essential oils in the recipe by half.

There is much controversy about using essential oils with those that have epilepsy or high blood pressure, although, there has not been much documentation done on essential oils causing problems with either. If you feel you should avoid certain essential oils, by all means, do so.

However, there is documentation that suggests strong odors or smells can sometimes trigger an epileptic seizure. If you are unsure one may want to avoid essential oils such as Eucalyptus globulus and Rosemary, other oils that may be included but are not limited to this list are Camphor and Tea Tree.

Before I forget, do not take essential oils internally. The term Aroma – Therapy means to smell the aromas for therapy. It does not say to swallow them ever (unless prescribed by a medical doctor).

Herbs are made for ingesting not essential oils. Moreover, this book is about "AROMA THERAPY" not herbs!

Essential oils should always be diluted if applying to the skin.

The old assumption that certain essential oils can be used directly (also known as "Neat" or "Neatly") on the skin should be revised.

Although Lavender and Tea Tree were once considered safe to use undiluted on the skin, just ask anyone that used to do so on a regular basis and now can **never** use those oils again due to the allergic reaction they have developed.

Only on rare occasions and only as a one-time application should you ever apply Lavender or Tea Tree to the skin undiluted. A small drop on a wound or burn one time may not cause any problems.

Repeated applications of undiluted essential oils used while the wound heals could have unpleasant side effects down the road.

Essential oils can burn delicate tissues. They should never be applied near the eyes or other mucous membranes.

Do not apply undiluted essential oils to mucous membranes (eyes, mouth, vagina, or rectum). Never apply to the eyes and use extreme caution if applying oils and lotions that contain essential oils near or around the eyes.

If you are unsure about using an essential oil, then do not use it.

Often times there are other essential oils that can be blended that can bring about the desired effect you are trying to achieve.

The main safety points are:

- Keep out of the reach of Children and Pets.
- Use essential oils sparingly. More is not better.
- Use half the amount on children and the elderly.
- Avoid using the photosensitive essential oils for several hours before going into the sun.
- Do not use undiluted on the skin, if in doubt do a skin test before using any oils.
- Do not ingest. (A water/essential oil mouth rinse or gargle is not ingesting. Ingestion means swallowing.)
- Do not use essential oils during the first three months of Pregnancy, then limit thereafter, if you are concerned.
- Use caution with strong smelling oils around those with epilepsy.
- Avoid using essential oils around the eyes and other mucous membranes.
- Check with your medical practitioner if you have any health concern and/or are taking prescription medicines.
- One special note about Cats and Essential oils: A cats liver cannot metabolize or break down most essential oils so if you own cats, use caution using essential oils around them. Keep a 'safe' room – one that does not have essential oils being used in it – and never apply essential oils to your cat.
- Never ever, apply essential oils to your cat.
- Follow directions for the amount used in a recipe, using more is not going to be helpful in aromatherapy.
- If certain oils are listed in a recipe, it is because they will give the best results for the blend.
- Sometimes you can substitute oils but you may or may not get the same results.
- Do not apply essential oils to mucous membranes – eyes, mouth, vagina or rectum.

Proceed carefully if you are –

- Pregnant, even though you use essential oils every-day in toothpaste etc you will want to use them in a lower dilution than a normal blend, especially if applied to the skin. Pregnant women skin can develop sensitivities more easily than when not pregnant.

- have high blood pressure, open wounds, rashes, epilepsy

- If you are taking prescription medications or homeopathic remedies, check with a Certified Aromatherapist or your health care practitioner.

- Always use a skin test before using an essential oil for the first time.

- For skin use - dilute essential oils in fixed or carrier oil such as almond, jojoba, grape seed etc.

- DO NOT APPLY NEATLY. It has been suggested in the past that Lavender and Tea Tree oils could be used undiluted on the skin – or what you may have heard is called 'neat'. Research has shown that doing so can cause adverse effects and eventually the individual may develop sensitivity to those oils unnecessarily.

- For foot and body baths dilute in the water.

- Know which oils are photosensitive, which means to avoid exposure to the sun (most citrus oils are unless they are steam distilled), and to avoid going into the sun for 4 hours AFTER application of one of those oils.

ALWAYS check with your medical practitioner if you have any medical conditions such as high blood pressure or heart disease, kidney or liver disease and if you are on prescription medications.

Aromatherapy is considered to be a complementary medicine and NOT to be used instead of your medical practitioner.

Essential oils are wonderful products of nature. When used safely, they will truly enhance your life and the lives of those around you. Enjoy!!

What is Toxic? Phototoxic?

Toxic – it is a pretty scary word and it should be!!

In aromatherapy, this is a very big consideration when it comes to essential oils. The two types of toxicities are ingestion and photo toxicity.

Not every essential oil is toxic since many of them are used for food and flavoring. You must remember though that essential oils are used in small quantities in foods and beverages.

The danger occurs if ingested in too large of quantities and then they can be lethal (fatal).

This is one main reason the bottles are labeled to keep essential oils OUT of the REACH of CHILDREN!!! Small amounts of certain essential oils if ingested by a child can potentially cause death.

As we always say – this is "AROMA" THERAPY meaning you need to inhale (breathe in) not ingest them.

What is Photo Toxicity? This can be very serious.

Photo Toxicity or Sensitization can cause the skin to have anywhere from a slight color change to serious deep and weeping burns.

There are a few essential oils when they are used on the skin, then exposed to sunlight or UV lights, (such as in a suntan bed) can cause these reactions.

The discoloration or sores may never heal or may heal extremely slowly.

What essential oils are we talking about? The following essential oils that can cause photosensitization or Photo-toxicity include:

Bergamot**, expressed (but not the FCF – Bergaptine free bergamot), Angelica ROOT, Caraway, Cassia, Cedarwood-Virginian, Cinnamon BARK, Cumin, Ginger, Grapefruit, Mandarin expressed, Orange expressed, Rue**, Verbena.

There may be others, but these listed are considered mild to moderate to Severe**. (They are not listed in any particular order in this list).

To avoid sensitization or phototoxic reactions, one should remember to avoid bright sunlight or use of tanning beds for 6 hours after using ANY essential oil on the skin but absolutely avoid for those listed above!

Again, the warnings or cautions are about USE ON THE SKIN or ingestion (eating), usually not when they are used by inhalation or diffusing of any essential oil.

If you make your own massage oils, lotions or use essential oils in soaps, shampoos or perfumes AND, if you use any of the known phototoxic essential oils - stay out of the sun and tanning beds. Better yet, just use essential oils known to be safe for use on the skin.

This caution is extremely important for massage therapists and other folks that may use essential oils mixed with lotions, creams, etc that are applied to their client's skin. Make sure they are not going to a tanning bed or out into the sun for several hours.

If you are unsure about an essential oils safety for use on the skin that will be exposed to sunlight or tanning beds – simply omit it from your products that will be used on the skin.

Essential oils are wonderful and safe – *when used properly.*

They are packed with lots of goodness in small amounts. Do not be afraid to use them. Just use them with respect!

NOT ALL OILS ARE CREATED EQUAL

Only pure essential oils should be used by everyone.

They may cost more than the synthetic, perfumed, potpourri, or the lab (synthetic) created oils.

There are many different things to consider besides the price when choosing essential oils.

When purchasing essential oils please look for the following information on the bottle:

For Example:

Common name i.e. Lavender

Latin name which will include the species and sometimes the chemo-type (subspecies), i.e. *Lavendula angustifolia*

The country of origin, i.e. Bulgaria

The extraction or distilled method i.e. Steam Distilled

The plant part, i.e. Flowers

In addition, sometimes you will see listed the quality of the cultivation such as farm, ethical, wild crafted or organic.

For Aromatherapy use, use only pure 100% therapeutic quality oils that should include most of the above information.

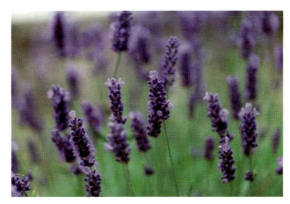

Lavender – *Lavendula angustifolia*

EDUCATION IS THE KEY

There are a several ways to learn about Aromatherapy.

One is to read, read and read some more. There are several good books out there to read and each author will give you just a little bit different approach (ways to use oils, different scenting of each oil).

Also, look for websites such as www.birchhillhappenings.com where the site is written by certified Aromatherapists that have been practicing for many years.

You can get books to help you for those beginning and for the intermediate and expert.

For beginners, start by getting a book that will use layman's terms explaining how to use essential oils and the cautions of the oils.

As you learn, you will develop a nose for aromatherapy.

By this, we mean start with 3 - 4 oils; get to know them by smell; how they are used, what properties they have and what oils can be blended. After you have gotten to 'know' those oils then add a few more and so on.

One more way of education is to take a home study course.

Start slowly by taking a class or a one-day workshop from Certified Aromatherapists.

As you will soon discover the study of Aromatherapy is a huge undertaking. You will learn in bits and pieces along the way.

Give yourself a lot of time to absorb all that you will learn. It will take years before you will feel comfortable in your knowledge to be able to share with your family and friends.

The benefit will be a more healthy life and emotionally stable sense of being.

HOW TO USE AROMATHERAPY

Some of the guidelines for using aromatherapy and the oils are very simple.

Follow the recipes and depend on the potency and precise concentration of the oils you may use only one or two drops.

So start by adding a drop or two. This is easy. Remember you cannot take a drop out but you can always add more if needed.

Inhalation (the BEST way) - start with 2 - 5 drops of essential oils. You can use a handkerchief, tissue or cotton ball. Ideally, a nasal inhaler is perfect. Do not smell straight from the bottle.

Clay or terra cotta diffusers - use 5 - 10 drops of essential oils. The heat of the room and sunlight will activate molecules and send the aromas into the room.

Room diffusion - use 10 - 15 drops of essential oils depending on the type and model of diffuser being used. There are fan diffusers, oil and wax tart warmers that can use either electricity or tea light for their heat source.

Body or Foot Bath - start with 2 - 5 drops of essential oils. Put drops into water after water has been drawn. Gently stir water to disperse oils.

Facial Steam - Start with 1 drop of essential oil in hot tap water, the water does not need to be boiling. Simply add 1 drop at a time, up to 5 drops to the hot water after pouring in bowl.

Stir gently to disperse the oils. Place towel over your head if desired, although this is usually not necessary. Place your face about 10" from water or wherever is comfortable.

Massage - Start with 15 drops of essential oils to 1 ounce of a fixed or carrier oil, or an unscented lotion for a body massage. Increase to 25 - 30 drops to 1 ounce for a targeted area. You can use up to 4 - 5 different essential oils in the massage blends.

Insect Repellant - Use 15 drops of essential oils to 1-ounce liquid such as distilled water or carrier oil, fractionated coconut oil is ideal.

One suggestion is to spray the repellant on your clothes if you are using the distilled water as your base liquid. You can apply it to all exposed areas of the body and reapply when necessary. Remember do not use photosensitive oils in the daylight hours.

Air Fresheners - Use 2 - 10 drops of essential oils to 1 ounce of water. Shake and spray into room to get rid of odors and to introduce enjoyable aromas.

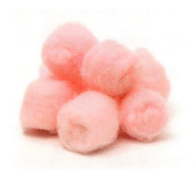

The simplest diffuser is a Cotton ball! Use a small bowl and put a few drops on the cotton. Gently inhale as desired.

A tea light diffuser uses either water or wax. Simply place your essential oils in the melted wax and light the candle. Soon you will smell the beautiful scenting.

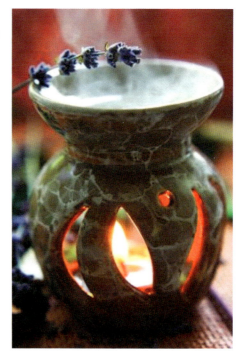

DIFFUSERS & DIFFUSING

There are many ways to diffuse the oils into the air.

One of the easiest is to place a few drops into a cotton ball and let the oils evaporate into the air.

Another way is a personal space diffuser using a specially designed clay or terra cotta diffusers. They are used the same way as the cotton balls.

Remember to use a glass, ceramic or stainless steel dish under your terra cotta or cotton balls. Essential oils should they leak through can do serious damage to finished surfaces. You do not want to damage your furniture.

Tart warmers are a very good way to diffuse essential oils.

You simply add a wax tart to the bowl, turn the diffuser on, when the wax has melted then add your oils, the heat of the wax will 'excite' the molecules of the oils and 'push' them into the air. You can reuse the wax tart over again by adding more essential oils.

Electric diffusers with a fan use a fiber pad or refill cartridge where you place 5 - 6 drops of oil(s) on the surface. The air (either being pushed through or pulled from the cartridge) will quickly diffuse the oils into the air. With this much air movement you will need to replenish the essential oils on the pad every 2-3 hours.

Nasal inhalers – these are small enough so you can carry them with you wherever you go. They are a very discreet way to use essential oils for specific ailments.

All you have to do is add a couple of drops of oil to the inside cotton pad. You can inhale whenever you need to.

Some of them are quite nice looking and no one will know you are using it as a way to use essential oils!

There are also diffuser lamps where a candle is used with either a glass or ceramic bowl above the candle.

One thing to consider before using a candle heated (Tea light) diffuser is there are no 'soot-free' candles.

Even so-called soot-free tea light candles will still produce burnt particles that will be floating in the air.

If you have any type of respiratory ailment you should choose another method of diffusion, not candle type diffusers.

To use the tea light diffuse you could pour water in the bowl with 3 - 4 drops of the oil(s) you are going to use. The heat of the candle will warm the water and disperse the aroma into the air.

Be careful as you don't want the flame from the candle to be too close to the bowl as the temperature of the flame is around 1800 degrees so if the flame is too close to the bowl you can 'burn' the oils and they won't smell nice.

DO NOT put more water to a hot bowl. Make sure it is cool enough to touch. For better control, we suggest you only use wax tarts in all heat or flame style diffusers.

Atomizers have a glass nebulizer part where you pour in the oils. The molecules of the oils are pushed into the air by a pump and the vibration of the nebulizer.

Some of the problems with atomizers will result in the nebulizer (glass part) to clog with oil and it is hard to clean them out. Only thin oils should be used with an atomizer type diffuser.

Recently there has been an influx of ultrasonic style diffusers. These too can easily become dysfunctional if you do not follow the manufacturer's instructions. Since these types of units are very expensive, please follow the directions and use only as directed.

Finally yet importantly, is one of our most favorite types of diffuser as it is used at the very most personal level. It is jewelry.

There are several types of jewelry (sterling silver, terra cotta for instance) now available so you can add a couple of drops of your favorite oil and have it near you when you want them.

This type of diffuser is handy for your very own therapeutic needs to help with any variety of emotional or mental stimulating aromatherapy need.

FOR THE BEGINNER

For those just starting out in Aromatherapy what do you need?

We suggest you purchase a couple of good books. There are dozens of good ones available.

For instance:

- Aromatherapy for Dummies by Kathi Keville.

- The Complete Book of Essential Oils and Aromatherapy by Valerie Ann Worwood.

- And for Aromatherapy Recipes don't forget Penny's book Aromatherapy Recipes using Pure Essential Oils Volume 1.

Then of course, you will need a few essential oils.

You can purchase them separately, such as lavender, peppermint, rosemary, ylang ylang or in a 'beginners' kit of some type.

You will want to get a few empty bottles - you just need small ones when you are just starting out.

You might need a few droppers too. If you purchase 4ml to 10 ml bottles of essential oils, they usually have a dropper insert in the top of the bottle to let one drop out at a time.

Small quantities may come just in the container with no insert. The oils will not come out as with the small quantity causes a vacuum to form and they cannot come out.

Essential oils should not be used directly on the skin.

All essential oils should be mixed properly before being used on the skin. Therefore, you will want a couple carrier or fixed oils too, such as Sweet Almond, jojoba, or grape seed oils.

You will also want to get some denatured alcohol or high proof vodka. This is used to clean your droppers and bottles of all traces of essential oil.

You do not want to contaminate your expensive oils by not cleaning your droppers between oils. Make sure the droppers are completely dry before you use them.

You might want to have some distilled water and a spray bottle for making room freshening mists.

You will need a diffuser to enjoy your newly created blends.

Once you are ready, you might want to try mixing them in unscented shampoos, conditioners or bath and shower gels.

Journaling is a very important part of Aromatherapy

As you begin learning about the uses of essential oils, you will find that keeping good records is necessary.

Whether you are a beginner or advanced – the best aroma therapists get to 'know' their oils and what they do for them and their clients by writing things down.

You have several methods you can do this: Simply keep a notebook (such as a '3' ring binder), a recipe card filing system or other file folder.

Today the options for keeping records are many. They can be handwritten or typed and printed from a computer, etc. Use the method you feel will be the most beneficial for you.

The next question is what records should I be keeping?

You will want to keep at least two types of records – One of the essential oil and one for the condition(s) you use it for. This will make quick references when the time comes for you to find out what worked for you previously.

Start with a set of records about the essential oils used. Things like its common name, botanical name and species, and country of origin. These are easily found on the bottle labels.
This important information should be listed on your bottles of essential oil.

Also, include on this card a record of the conditions or ailments you used it for and the results you received/achieved.

A simple example would be:
Eucalyptus – Eucalyptus globulus, Australia:
Used for:
Chest congestion – It worked great for me when inhaled but Bob did not appear to respond as well (but he did better with

Eucalyptus – Eucalyptus radiata – (see that entry)
Muscle soreness – Bob overworked this weekend – made a massage blend with Sweet Almond oil in a 3% dilution and it worked great!

Then on another set of cards will be your "Conditions".

You will want to make an Entry or Card for *Chest Congestion* and one for *Muscle Soreness.* Writing down the essential oils you used at the time and the results for the individuals, you used on them. This helps you remember exactly what you used and how you applied it.

Your Chest Congestion card might look like this:
Chest Congestion:
Eucalyptus globulus - worked on me. I inhaled it using a personal inhaler.
Eucalyptus radiata: gave Bob relief when used in a steam bowl.

Your Muscle Soreness card might look like this:
Muscle Soreness:
Due to overworked muscles:
Eucalyptus globulus: 3% dilution with Sweet almond oil.
Peppermint (Mentha piperita): 2% dilution in Jojoba
Recipe:
Eucalyptus globulus – 3 drops
Peppermint (Mentha piperita) – 3 drops
Sunflower oil - 1 tablespoon (This is a 2% dilution of essential oils to Carrier oil)

This is just a simple way for you to remember what did and did not work for that given situation. More importantly, what were essential oils can do for you for a certain ailment or condition.

Before long, your list of properties for each individual essential oil will become very long.

You will soon find out why in aromatherapy when someone asks you what 'such and such' essential oil is good for – you will most likely answer the same as we do. "There are too many to list."

And then, we add....
"But what condition are you having problems with? Maybe we can find a few essential oils that will work for you!"

As you continue to use and study essential oils, your file folder or notebook will be the best guide for you and your family. It will be your own personal Aromatherapy book of reference! Moreover, it will be what works best for you!

FIRST – LEARNING HOW TO SMELL ESSENTIAL OILS

Everyone wants to smell the wonderful (and not to wonderful) scents of essential oils but most people smell them wrong or just haven't been instructed on the best and proper way to smell them.

They want to smell them directly out of the bottle. This is a big "No-No". This is not the correct way to smell essential oils at all.

So please do not smell out of the bottle or the cap.

The proper way is to place 1-2 drops on a perfumers Scent Testing Strips or blotter. Of course, if you do not have any then you can use an unscented tissue or paper towel.

Write down on each strip or paper the name of the oils you will be dropping on that particular strip.

To avoid sensory overload we suggest you smell no more than 5-6 oils at one sitting. More than this and your sense of smell may block all the scents and you will not be able to continue.

In addition, you risk making yourself ill. Even though essential oils are natural and most of the time very pleasant, trying to smell too many at one time can upset your system.

You will want to smell the various essential oils in intervals. Turn your head away from the strip or tissue, take a breath in and exhale.

Then place the strip under your nose about 3-5 inches away and take in a short light whiff. Do not inhale deeply.

Make a note of what it smells such as fruity, herb like, wood like, spicy, earthy, etc.

You can use any description you like as long as you make a note for future reference.

The next sniff or whiff you can smell a little more deeply. Again, write down your notes.

Then before you are done, you will take one more sniff.

This time you will want to puff a little warm air from your nose onto the pad (just a small puff) and then inhale again.

The warming will often bring about other scents you may not have known existed. This is especially true when you are comparing synergy blends.

If you are smelling blends, and as you continue to 'sniff your whiffs' you may be able to pick out the individual oils in each blend!

In addition, if you are inhaling single essential oils they may change over time and have a different slightly different odor.

Now wait five minutes and take another smell. You can do the short whiff or the longer slow smell. Again, write down your smells.

You can continue to sniff after 15, 30 minutes and 1 hour. You can decide how long you want to continue to smell the oils. You should smell again 24 hours later to really get to know them.

Most oils will be totally gone or evaporated after that long. Some though will not. Some may linger for a week or longer. Write this down. This information is very helpful if you decide to become interested in making your own perfumes or body scenting.

Remember the 'Lock and Key' of your brain will help you to remember the scents for future identification.

The next time you smell one of your blends and you have locked into memory the various smell of a wide variety of essential oils (one or more) in that blend will quickly be identified.

OH NO – I CAN'T SMELL THE OILS – WHAT HAPPENED?
What is Olfactory Fatigue?

Everyone loves to smell essential oils. Diffusing essential oils can make for a very pleasant and wonderful smelling room, but if you put too much or too little oil into the air pretty soon you cannot smell them.

The oils are still in the air – cleaning, disinfecting and scenting, but as you stay in the room, you may no longer smell the oil.

What happened? Well, your body and olfactory sensors have become accustomed to the smell. You have what is called 'Olfactory fatigue'. The olfactory senses have blocked the smell of that particular scent.

What is "OLFACTORY FATIGUE"? This is a very normal body response with the sense of smell.

It is a part of your primordial brain. It involves the "Fright and Flight" response of animals and 'humans' too. Your nose constantly smells the air for 'threats'. For most humans your nose smells for fire, burned toast or food, skunks or other stinky smells. However, wild animal noses are searching smells for other predators. Just ask any hunter – why do they want to stay 'down wind" when they are hunting? You got it; they do not want the animal to know they are hunting to smell them. Wilds animals will usually smell humans as a threat.

Just realize your nose and body cannot tell the difference (threat wise) between a sweet smelling essential oil and a fire.

AFTER your brain has determined that the essential oils or the smell of smoke is not a threat – your senses of smell will then BLOCK that odor. You will not be able to smell the essential oil nor the smoke after anywhere from 5-30 minutes depending on how quickly your brain will dismiss the smell as a threat.

Unless you leave the building for several minutes, (your nose usually needs at least 15 minutes) to reset your sense of smell, you will not be able to smell them again. Nevertheless, just like before – once your brain determines it is not a threat your sense of smell will block it again. This time and each subsequent time, it will block the smells more quickly.

As stated above, to smell the scent again you will need to 'reset' your sense of smell. Simply leave the room for 15-30 minutes – step out doors and get some fresh air if possible.

When you re-enter the room you will smell the scent again. If not, maybe you do need to add more essential oils to your diffuser.

We know there are those whose sense of smell will block the scent out within 10 -15 minutes. It is possible even *your brain* will again block the smell and you will think the oils are all gone.

There is nothing wrong with you, just your sense of smell getting used to the scents or odors that are present.

Do not add more scenting until you have performed the "leave the room" test. Once you have done the test and if you smell the scent, again you will not necessarily need to add more.

Doing the 'leave the room test' is to prevent the potential to overdose or over use the oils. Just realize they are there but you just cannot smell them due to olfactory fatigue (unless you leave the room and re-enter later).

Even if you cannot smell them but very faintly, the essential oils are still there doing their thing whether it be for physical, psychological or spiritual needs.

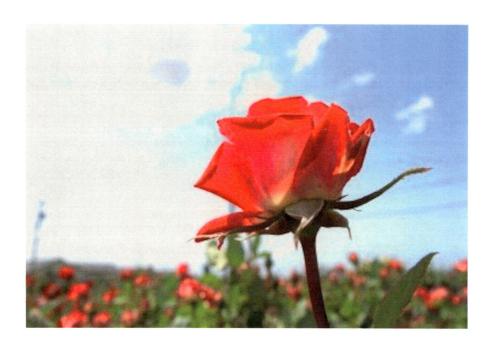

WHAT OILS SHOULD YOU BEGIN WITH?

A nice beginner kit may include Bergamot, Clary sage, Eucalyptus, Grapefruit, Lavender, Lemon, Peppermint, Rosemary, Tea Tree and Ylang ylang, or any combination of these most commonly used essential oils.

Once you have really become familiar with each of the oils you will want to add more. You will soon have your favorites and will want to experiment with more. Therefore, you may want some of the large variety of essential oils available.

Always buy a small quantity of an essential oil at first. For the majority of essential oils, until you really have a need for them, buy a 'working' sample. Many companies will offer 'sniff' samples but they are not in quantities you can accurately smell.

They may not help you to 'get to know' that oils scent.

In addition, since essential oils can be quite costly, you do not want oils just sitting around if you do not like them.

Moreover, if you do not need them now they many deteriorate before you use them.

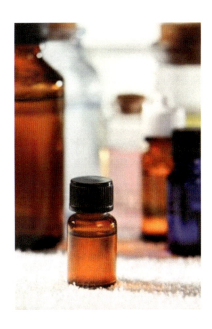

SOME COMMON OILS - THEIR PROPERTIES AND USES

Following are ten of the most commonly used essential oils and are an excellent choice for the beginner. Included will be just a few of the many properties and uses each essential oil has been traditional known to be useful.

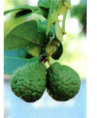

Bergamot - *Citrus bergamia* – is a light greenish-yellow in color, with a fruity-spicy aroma, uplifting and refreshing.

Uses: acne, cold sores, eczema, loss of appetite, sore throat, cystitis, colds and flu, depression, anxiety and stress related conditions.

Properties – analgesic, antiseptic, antidepressant, carminative, digestive, parasiticide, tonic, antispasmodic

Blends with - lavender, neroli, jasmine, cypress, geranium, lemon, chamomile, juniper berry, cedarwood, clary sage, coriander, geranium, frankincense, rose, sandalwood and vetiver

CAUTION: this is a phototoxic essential oil. Do not use on skin that will be exposed to sunlight or tanning beds. It will cause a chemical type burn and damage to the skin. This oil is best used in a diffuser if there is any risk of being exposed to sunlight within 4 hours of use on the skin.

IF you need to use for skin applications then purchase Bergamot FCF. It has had the Furo-Coumarin removed and will be safe to use in sun.

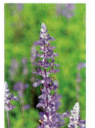

Clary sage - *Salvia sclarea* - pale yellow with a spicy, herbaceous, camphorous aroma with a floral under note.

Uses - dandruff, depression, energy (lack of), exhaustion (nervous), oily hair and skin, muscle aches, stress, migraine, inflammation

Properties - anti-inflammatory, antimicrobial, antiseptic, antispasmodic, cicatrisant, digestive, diuretic, emmenagogue, stomachic, tonic

Blends with - bergamot, cypress, frankincense, geranium, grapefruit, jasmine, juniper berry, lavender, lemon, lime, neroli, orange, petitgrain, pine and sandalwood

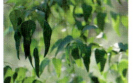

Eucalyptus - *Eucalyptus globulus* – is a colorless with a strong camphorous aroma with a woody undertone. It is head clearing and cooling.

Uses - asthma, bronchitis, coughs, fever, headache, lung infections, pneumonia, sinus problems, rheumatism, urinary tract infections, viral infections, muscular aches and pains

Properties - analgesic, anti-rheumatic, antiseptic, antiviral, antispasmodic, decongestant, diuretic, expectorant, rubefacient, stimulant, vermifuge and vulnerary

Blends with - rosemary, lavender, thyme, marjoram, pine, cedarwood and lemon

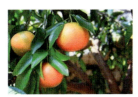

Grapefruit - *Citrus paradisi* – the color can vary depending on the source of the essential oil, from an orange, to yellow or greenish color with a sweet crisp, citrus aroma

Uses - acne, anorexia, cellulite, colds, depression, headache, jet lag, sore and tires muscles, oily skin and hair, stress, tinea and tiredness

Properties - antiseptic, antitoxic, astringent, bactericidal, diuretic, stimulant (lymphatic and digestive) and tonic

Blends with - lemon, bergamot, palmarosa, rosemary, cypress, lavender, geranium and other spice oils

Caution: this oil will oxidize and deteriorate and is best used within one year of harvest if it is to be used on the skin.

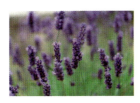

Lavender - *Lavandula angustifolia* - also known as the "Mother" of all oils, is a colorless to pale yellow, with a sweet, floral-herbaceous aroma that is uplifting, refreshing and calming.

Uses - burns, cellulite, cough, dermatitis, slow digestion, flatulence, headache, insect bites, insomnia, psoriasis, scars, sprains, sunburn, tension and wounds

Properties - analgesic, antibacterial, antidepressant, antimicrobial, anti-rheumatic, antiseptic, antispasmodic, carminative, cholagogue, emmenagogue, insecticide, nervine, sedative, stimulant, stomachic, vulnerary

Blends with - most oils, especially floral and citrus, cedarwood, clove, clary sage, pine, geranium, juniper berry, rose and patchouli

Lemon - *Citrus limonum* - pale yellow with a light uplifting and refreshing citrus scent

Uses - acne, brittle nails, slow circulation, herpes, indigestion, infection, influenza, liver - congestion, mouth ulcers, sore throat, varicose veins, warts

Properties - antimicrobial, antiseptic, antitoxic, astringent, bactericidal, carminative, insecticidal, stimulates white blood cells, tonic, and vermifuge

Blends with - lavender, ylang ylang, rose, sandalwood, frankincense, chamomile, fennel, geranium, eucalyptus, juniper and other citrus oils

Caution: this is a phototoxic essential oil. Do not use on skin that will be exposed to sunlight or tanning beds within 4 hours of application to the skin. As with other citrus essential oils, the shelf life is about 1 year.

Peppermint - *Mentha piperita* - pale yellow with a high minty camphorous aroma that is highly penetrating to the nasal passages. It is bright, energizing and head clearing.

Uses - asthma, bronchitis, catarrh, colon - spastic, cramps, diarrhea, exhaustion, fever, flatulence, headache, heartburn, hysteria, indigestion, intestinal parasites, mental fatigue, muscle pain, nausea, shock, vertigo, worms

Properties – analgesic, anti-inflammatory, antimicrobial, antiseptic, antispasmodic, antiviral, astringent, carminative, cholagogue, decongesting, expectorant, febrifuge, nervine, stomachic and vermifuge

Blends with - rosemary, lavender, marjoram, lemon, eucalyptus clary sage, geranium and other mints

Caution: this essential oil is very concentrated. Start with just a drop or two when blending. A little may overpower your blend.

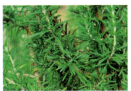

Rosemary - *Rosmarinus officinalis* – is a colorless or pale yellow with a refreshing, head clearing, minty-herbaceous aroma and a camphorous undertone.

Uses - acne, baldness, burns, circulation - slow, dermatitis, fatigue, gout, headache, lice, muscular pains, myalgia, mental fatigue, psoriasis, rheumatism, scabies, sciatica, sinusitis, tinea, varicose veins, whooping cough

Properties - analgesic, antimicrobial, antioxidant, antiseptic, cephalic, diuretic, nervine, parasitic, stimulant, tonic and vulnerary

Blends with - lavender, citronella, citrus oils, oregano, thyme, pine, basil, peppermint, elemi, cedarwood, petitgrain, cinnamon and other spice oils

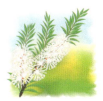

Tea Tree - *Melaleuca alternifolia* - pale yellow or clear color with fresh spicy-camphorous aroma

Uses - acne, asthma, athletes foot, boils, bunions, coughs, cracked skin, dermatitis, eczema, flu, fleas, fungal infection, gingivitis, insect bites and stings, lice, lung infections, muscular aches, psoriasis, rheumatism, ringworm, sore throat, thrush, vaginal infections, warts, wounds

Properties - anti-infectious, anti-inflammatory, antiseptic, antiviral, bactericidal, expectorant, fungicidal, germicidal, immune-stimulant, parasiticide, vulnerary

Blends with - clary sage, clove, eucalyptus, geranium, lemon, lavender, marjoram, nutmeg, rosemary, pine and spice oils

Ylang ylang - *Cananga odorata* - pale yellow with a sweet, floral, spicy aroma. Ylang ylang is also known as the 'flower of flowers'.

Uses - acne, aphrodisiac, depression, skin, hair growth, hair rinse, headache, insect bites, insomnia, muscle aches, scars, stress, wounds

Properties - anti-allergic, antibacterial, antidepressant, antifungal, anti-inflammatory, antimicrobial, antiseptic, antispasmodic, antiviral, aphrodisiac, cell proliferant, disinfectant, expectorant, germicidal, nervine, sedative, vulnerary

Blends with - balsam, bergamot, jasmine, rose, rosewood, vetiver

FIXED and CARRIER OILS

When making massage oils or blends for use on the skin you will need to use fixed carrier oil.

They are oils that have been cold pressed or expeller pressed from any variety of plants nuts and seeds.

Commonly used are Sweet Almond, Apricot kernel, Grapeseed, Fractionated Coconut and other Coconut oils, Jojoba just to name a few.

There are many other oils that are used for massage or for specific skin conditions.

Carrier oils do not have an odor such as the essential oils and they do not evaporate.

However, they are subject to oxidation and have shelf life of around 2 years with the exception of the Coconut oils and Jojoba.

Coconut oils and jojoba have a much longer shelf life at 5 years. Although it is quite rare that these would ever be sitting around that long since they are very popular oils.

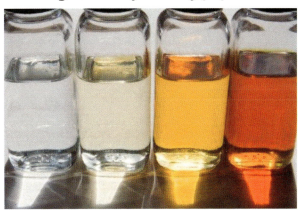

Carrier oils – vary in color depending on the plant source.

Left to right:
Fractionated Coconut oil, Virgin Coconut oil, Sweet Almond and Rosehip seed oil.

SHELF LIFE OF ESSENTIAL OILS AND FIXED OILS

Most essential oils have a shelf life of 2 to 5 years and several have a shelf life of well over 5 years, but then there are those that are pretty much expired when they are even less than 2 years old. Thankfully, there are just a handful of those.

No essential oil though has to be tossed out even if you know it is past its therapeutic effective shelf life. You can always use them for cleaning, freshening and scenting. They may not be as potent at killing germs or fungus but will still be able to disinfect to varying degrees.

In Therapeutic Aromatherapy, essential oils used to treat any ailment or condition should be the freshest oils you can purchase. Alternatively, they should definitely fall within the 2-5 years since being purchased if that is their shelf life. Other factors can determine if your oils are still in the therapeutic ranges.

The majority of essential oils fall in the 2-5 year shelf life. Nevertheless, many factors can shorten the shelf life. Moreover, they have to do with storage and use. Number '1 and 2' – Keep them tightly capped and Keep them cool!

If you buy a larger bottle of essential oils, you should not leave the cap off while you are blending. Keep it shut except when measuring it out.

Also, as your essential oils become less in each bottle – transfer them into smaller bottles to reduce the headspace so less air and oxygen is in the bottle.

Too much headspace can further deteriorate your oils. Oxidation will destroy most essential oils and each time your bottle is opened new oxygen enters it. Combine that with heat and your oils will deteriorate very quickly.

Citrus and Pine essential oils have the shortest life span. They should be replaced every 12 months if you are using them for any health ailment.

Citrus oils that are used for uplifting and alertness need to be fresh. Pine oils used for congestion and upper respiratory ailments need to be fresh too.

Do not use old Citrus or Pine oils on the skin as they age because some of the constituents become strong skin sensitizers and could cause unwanted rashes or other problems. They can still be used for scenting. They can still be used in mop buckets too, but may not have the disinfecting properties as when they are under a year of age.

As for essential oils that have long shelf lives usually, they are the thicker ones, such as Cedarwood, Sandalwood, Patchouli, Vetiver and a few others.

Exception to this thick oil quality will be the essential oil of Rose Otto. Rose Otto gets better too with age – BUT only if it is kept in a cool, dark place with little headspace. If not, it too will lose many of its wonderful properties. Worse yet, Rose Otto is so volatile it will easily evaporate out of a tightly capped bottle unless kept refrigerated.

As for carrier oils, the majority have a shelf life of around 2 years when stored in the refrigerator. They will start to go rancid even earlier if not kept in a cool place also.

Some carrier oils such as Borage and Evening Primrose are extremely susceptible to oxidations and after 6-8 months will need to be tossed. Keep these refrigerated and tightly capped in a bottle. If you should need to add these to a blend or skin formulation, we suggest you purchase some that are in the soft gel capsules and use those in your blend. They are less likely to have gone rancid, provided they were refrigerated.

The EXCEPTIONS to carrier oil are for Jojoba (which is really a liquid wax) and the Coconut oils – Virgin, Expeller pressed or Fractionated. The latest research shows each of those oils have well over 5 years shelf life. Therefore, our suggestions are the following:

If you have essential oils older than 2 years sitting on your shelf and are, using them for THERAPEUTIC aromatherapy set them aside and buy fresh for your therapeutic needs. Use the OLDER oils for cleaning and scenting realizing they may not possess all the properties as a more fresh oil would.

If you use carrier oils for massage and they are not Jojoba or one of the Coconut oils then you should throw them away after 1 year of sitting on your shelf. The carrier oils may have gone rancid and even though the essential oils added to them may have a longer shelf life, the essential oils will not extend the life of the carrier oil.

Contrary to common practices by many folks, adding Wheat Germ oil or Vitamin E as a preservative WILL NOT work. Both, Wheat germ oil or Vitamin E, are ineffective preservatives for carrier oils as both will go rancid very quickly and due to their odor will alter the finished products!

Best Advice: Buy smaller quantities of essential oils and carrier oils that can be used up each year!

Just remember as good as it is to have a large variety of essential oils and carrier oils on hand, you need to take stock of your inventory.

Write dates on the bottle when you open them up and try to use them within 1 year of opening or better yet purchasing, to get the most therapeutic use of your valuable essential oils.

Buy in small quantities so you can always use 'fresh' oils that will give you the best results when used in therapeutic applications.

Do not expect oil that has sat on your shelf for 3 years or more to provide the same therapeutic actions as one that is less than a year old.

The old adage –"If in doubt, throw it out" applies to essential oils and carrier oils too. If you do not know how long ago you purchased the oil, you are better off getting a new bottle than having poor results from one that is too old.

BLENDING
When blending your essential oils remember to measure carefully. Most of the time you will be measuring drops of essential oils.

Almost all recipes are given by numbers of drops that are added. Many recipes are proportional - meaning that if a recipe calls for 5 drops of this oil, 3 drops of that oil, you can always mix 5 ml of this oil and 3 ml of that oil. This way you can make larger 'batches' easily and still have the same blend.

If you are trying to mix your essential oils in with water based ingredients or in water, you may need to first mix it with an Emulsifier

An emulsifier is anything that will allow you to mix oil and water. Common products are coconut emulsifier, perfumers' alcohol, Polysorbate 20, 60 or 80, turkey red castor oil to name a few. These will help the essential oils to blend with your water-based products.

When mixing essential oils with carrier oils for use in massage you should never make a stronger blend than 2-3%.

How to figure out how much is in a 2% or 3% solution? First, think of things in drops. If you have 100 drops of something, you would have a 2 percent solution if 2 drops were an essential oil and 98 drops were the carrier oil. Another way to measure it would be 2 ml of essential oil and 98 ml of the carrier oil.

Looking at the first example: 2 drops of Essential oil - that is easy. However, the 98 drops of carrier oil that is not so easy, but you can do a little more math and convert the drops into teaspoons. Since there are about 20 drops per ml and 5 ml per teaspoon, you can easily figure it out. 98 divided by 20 is approximated 5. You have 5 ml or 1 teaspoon (or 98-100 drops of carrier oil).

A 2% solution would be 2 drops essential oil per teaspoon of carrier oil 3% would be 3 drops per teaspoon.

Some essential oils work better when mixed with different carrier oils. If you see your essential oils not mixing with particular carrier oil, you will have to experiment with other carrier oils.

Some essential oils and absolutes will become 'saturated' in the carrier oil. When this occurs, you cannot get any more essential oil or absolute to mix in with the carrier oil.

You will see it initially being in solution, but if you let it set for a day or two, you will either see the absolute sitting on the bottom, or the essential oil sitting on the top of your carrier oil.

Actually, this can happen with any unscented base product used. Shampoos, conditioners, and lotions are all prone to having the essential oil separate out. (Did you remember to use an emulsifier for your shampoo or bottle of water in your spray mister?)

Simply shake, or stir your bottle of product to mix the essential oils back into the product before using. Actually, shaking your blends a little before using is a good thing to do to redistribute your essential oils in the product.

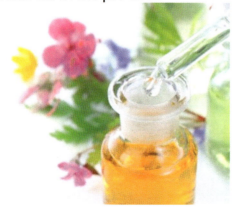

There are a few essential oils when blended together that will not mix or they actually will cause a chemical reaction and become a solid chunk of 'goo' in the bottom of your bowl, bottle or jar. Fortunately, this is rare.

Do not let anything stop you from being creative. Essential oils are oils composed of several different chemical constituents. When mixed together you will sometimes see them get cloudy, then add another essential oil and the mixture will become clear. Sometimes the blend will cause sediment to form.

These are normal reactions when you mix certain essential oils together. Even though you are not a chemist, you will eventually observe these reactions when blending different oils or when making up our blends.

Next: Store your custom blends of essential oils in glass bottles. Be sure to put labels on them with the essential oils you used. You will be able to use a drop or two without having to mix it fresh each time you want to enjoy your favorite blend.

Remember to only mix as much as you will use in 4-6 months. You always want to try to use the freshest blends and essential oils.

When mixing massage or bath blends we suggest you mix the essential oils together first before you add the carrier oil. Then let the mixture "age" or blend for several days before using.

Remember also that pure essential oils will disintegrate rubber and certain types of plastic materials. Never leave your bottles stopped with rubber bulb capped droppers. In just a few days, the rubber will be a terrible blob of black goo!

To blend essential oils with carrier oils you can mix them in PET plastic bottles or Glass bottles. PET plastic bottles will not deteriorate when used with essentials oils, other types of plastic bottles may.

MEASURING, PERCENTAGES, HOW MUCH?

These subjects are all related and are asked about many times each month. Therefore, we felt it was time to review these.

When you are making massage oils or scenting lotion or creams knowing how to measure, figure percentages and how much is safe to add are important to know.

For general everyday use, essential oils are measured in milliliters and drops. In big industry, they are measured by weight. Most of us that make just a few blends for your own personal use do not need to invest in scales that can weigh in milligrams.

Here are a few charts to help you.

Metric Measure	Decimal for fluid ounces	Common Fraction for fluid ounces	By drops (approximate due to viscosity of each essential oil)
1 mL	0.0335 fl oz	1 /30 fl oz	20-25
2 mL	0.067 fl oz	1/15 to 1/16 fl oz	40-50
4 mL	0.135 fl oz	1/8 fl oz (approximately)	80-100
5 mL	0.169 fl oz	1/6 fl oz	100-125
10 mL	0.33 fl oz	1/3 fl oz	Drops should not be
15 mL	0.5 fl oz	1/2 fl oz	counted for blending
29.573 mL	1 fl oz	1 fl oz	large amounts of
30 mL	1.014 fl oz	1 fl oz	essential oils therefore
50 mL	1.69 fl oz	1 2/3 fl oz	no drop values for these
60 mL	2 28 fl oz	2 fl oz	have been listed.

To make blends of products by percentages here is a handy chart showing the number of drops to add to the volume of your finished products. You can use this for blending massage oils, shampoos, lotion or creams etc.

When you are blending massage oils and lotions, you will need to know how much to add to your finished product to be at a safe therapeutic level. Below is a chart to help you easily know how many drops to add to various volumes of your finished product.

Total Volume of finished product	1%	2%	4%
1 tablespoon	3 drops	6 drops	12 drops
1 oz (2 tablespoons)	6 drops	12 drops	24 drops
2 oz (4 TBS)	12 drops	24 drops	48 drops or ½ tsp.
4 oz (1/2 cup)	24 drops	48 drops (½ tsp.)	96 drops (1 tsp.)
8 oz (1 cup)	48 drops (½ tsp.)	96 drops (1 tsp.)	10 ml or 2 tsp.
16 oz (2 cup)	96 drops (1 tsp.)	10 ml (2 tsp.)	20 ml (4 tsp.)

Remember to use essential oils safely always use ½ the amounts for children and the elderly that you would use for an adult.

In other words if your recipe is a 3% blend for normal adults, you should make a 1% or 1½% blend for children, etc.

Add the number of drops of essential oils to your blending container then fill the container with the volume of the base product listed on the left. Mix well and let sit for 24 hours before use if possible.

 The general rule of thumb in aromatherapy is to use a 2% dilution of essential oils when added to any finished product that is to be applied to the skin. Of course, there are exceptions.

The simple thing to remember about adding essential oil to your final product is if the final product is going to remain on the skin the essential oils in the blend should be about a 2% dilution (or less if used on a baby or the elderly).

If your blend is going to be used in a product that will be washed off or rinsed away, you can blend it stronger – up to a 5-10% dilution although this is not usually necessary.

Products that are washed off or rinsed away include Shampoos, Hair Conditioners, & Shower gel.

Lotion or products used on and left on the skin such as toners and massage oils should only be blended in a 1% or 2% dilution, again less if used on babies or the elderly.

Here are some general guidelines:

Mixed with lotion, creams or massage oils – 6 drops per ounce of carrier base

Shampoos, Hair Conditioners, & Shower gel. – 10-12 drops per ounce of product

Essential oils can be added to distilled water for use on the skin, such as a toner – 3-4 drops essential oils per ounce of water.

Used in a Facial Steam – no more than 5 drops of essential oils to 2 cups of hot water.

Room spray – added to distilled water or other water base for spraying – Varies with the essential oils used. It is not unusual for it to be as high as 50 drops of essential oils per 4 ounces of water.

You should use an emulsifier when you are blending essential oils and a water-based product.

We hope this will help you decide on how much to use in your blends.

As always, if you should develop any kind of irritation, then you should discontinue use and reformulate your recipe for next time. Also, start with less essential oil and only add more to your blends as needed.

SUPPLIES

Some supplies you may need are:

Small glass bottles for storing such as 4ml and 10ml with caps and orifice reducers to get drops out

Glass bottles in 1oz and 2oz

PET (plastic) bottles in 2, 4 and 8oz sizes with disc or spray tops

Pipettes and droppers

Beakers and stirring rods

Glass liquid measuring cups with pour spouts

Stainless steel measuring spoons

Wire whip or French whisks

Larger glass or stainless steel bowls – do not use plastic

Paper towels

CLEANING YOUR GLASSWARE

After a busy day of blending or if you wish to reuse your essential oil bottles you will need to clean them thoroughly.

Use the hottest water available and some soap or detergent. Let them soak for a few minutes. Use a small bottle or baby nipple cleaning brush to clean the insides, especially if you need to remove sediment. In tiny bottles, you can use a Q-tip or toothpick to remove stubborn remnants.

Rinse with more hot water, and turn upside down to drain on clean paper towels.

You are not done yet though, as you still could have a little bit of essential oil residue left inside your bottles or droppers.

The last thing to do is to rinse them with alcohol. We do not recommend rubbing or denatured alcohol as they have too much water content and other impurities in them. You can use high "proof" cheap vodka. It is virtually odorless and has no impurities.

The alcohol dissolves and helps remove any residual essential or carrier oils that might be in your bottles and droppers.

Using alcohol as the final rinse will help your glassware to dry quickly, enabling you to be able to store them away for your next blending session.

Do not try to clean anything that is made of plastic as essential oils quickly permeate this and make it nearly impossible to remove scents.

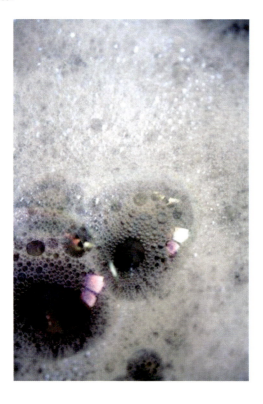

Essential Oil and Their Recipes have more than one use. Yes, Really They Do!

Mother Nature is so versatile and the plants and animals she provides have so many uses in our daily lives.

Just think about a tree for example. It can be used to build a home or furniture or eating utensils. It can be used for fuel to heat homes and businesses. If left in its natural state, they can provide shade in the summer. Not to mention how lovely it looks in your yard or the forest. In addition, the flowers, leaves, twigs, bark and roots might be used to make those wonderful essential oils!

Essential oils are no different. They have many different properties or uses. All are germicidal to varying degrees whether it is for viruses, bacteria or fungi.

Then they each possess a large variety of physical, emotional and spiritual properties. This helps them to be used in so many different applications.

So when you are looking for a recipe for a problem whether it is for an illness or ailment, be sure to use a good reference book that lists the various properties of essential oils too.

As an example, if you need a blend or recipe that has good decongestant properties and you know that Eucalyptus Globulus can do that really well. Look for a blend or create a new one that has Eucalyptus Globulus.

Sometimes you will find a recipe title that suggests it is for cleaning out the trash bin. Realize that recipe may work great for your congestion!

Remember and realize that the essential oils in that blend, although good for cleaning out the trash bin, also have some great essential oils to help with congestion. Blend it up and use it for congestion.

Most all recipes can be easily adapted for use in other applications.

An example here: you find a great massage blend you really love the smell of and would like to diffuse it in the bedroom, all you do is simply blend just the essential oils together in a glass bottle, omit the carrier oils or lotion and use in any diffuser.

Essential oils are so versatile and you being so creative can use many of these base recipes to have fun and a healthier and happier family and home.

Have fun, enjoy and most of all be creative!

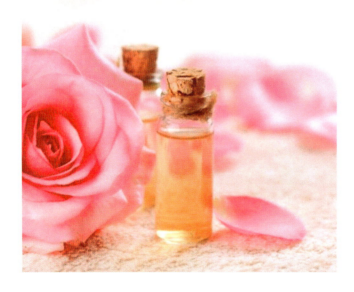

BLENDS TO TRY

Calming Massage oil

This blend is especially good after a hard day's work or work out at the gym.

Birch - 3 drops
Pine - 5 drops
Eucalyptus - 5 drops
Roman Chamomile - 3 drops
Sunflower oils - 2 ounces

Blend oils together, and then shake well. Massage into stiff tired muscles and simple enjoy and relax.

Massage oil for Sore Muscles

Ginger 2 drops
Cinnamon 4 drops
Cajuput 3 Drops
Chamomile 3 drops
15 ml of your favorite carrier oil

Mix all oils, and use as you would any massage oil. Work into muscles especially after a strenuous workout

Mood elevating bath

Rosewood (bois de rose) - 5 drops
Palmarosa - 5 drops
Grapefruit - 3 drops
Petitgrain - 2 drops
Carrier oil of your choice - 5ml

Blend in an amber bottle and shake. Put 4-6 drops of blend into a nice warm bath and enjoy.

Room disinfectant for diffusers
Pine - 6 drops
Cinnamon - 6 drops
Juniper - 5 drops
Clove - 3 drops

Blend in a glass bottle. Put 3 to 4 drops of blend in a diffuser or in an atomizer put 1ml or about 20 drops in.

Stress relief massage blend

Bergamot - 5 drops
Mandarin - 4 drops
Lavender - 4 drops
Nutmeg - 4 drops
Lemongrass - 3 drops
Carrier oil - 20ml

Blend in a glass bottle and shake to mix blend. Let sit for a day, then relax and either give the massage or be the recipient of the massage. Both of you will reap the benefits of the blend.

Refreshing Foot Bath

Rosemary - 6 drops
Lavender - 4 drops
Peppermint – 2 drops
Tea tree – 1 drop

Fill a basin with warm water and add the essential oils. Soak your feet for 10 – 15 minutes, adding more warm water if needed and enjoy.

Carpet Freshener

Eucalyptus – 30 drops
Cinnamon - 30 drops
Lemongrass - 30 drops
Clove bud - 10 drops
1/2 cup bicarbonate of soda (baking soda)

Blend all oils and soda in a wide mouth jar and close lid and let set for 24 hours. Sprinkle over carpet and let sit for 10-15 minutes then vacuum.

Foot Deodorizing Powder

Sage - 2 drops
Coriander - 2 drops
Spearmint - 2 drops
Talc powder - 2 ounce
Baking soda -1 tablespoon

Open the bottle of talc powder and add the baking soda. Shake well. Then add the drops of essential oil to a cotton pad or ball and drop inside the talc/baking soda bottle. Shake well and let sit for a couple days before using.

Dry Skin Formula

Jojoba - 1 teaspoon
Camellia - 1 teaspoon
Sesame - 1 teaspoon
Carrotseed essential oil - 25 drops
Sandalwood - 6 drops
Neroli - 4 drops
Geranium - 2 drops

Blend all ingredients in a 1 oz bottle; shake well to mix.
Apply 4 to 6 drops of blend twice a day to dry area.

Calming Diffuser Blend

Roman Chamomile - 20 drops
Lavender - 15 drops
Clary Sage - 10 drops
Geranium - 10 drops
Ylang ylang - 5 drops

Blend oils in a glass bottle and add to diffuser as needed.

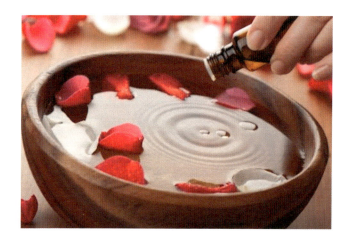

SOME HINTS

Remember –

More is not the case with Aromatherapy. Use the drops suggested or listed in a blend.

Be careful when going outside after using most citrus oils – many of them are phototoxic or photosensitive – which may cause discoloration of the skin.

In a car - use the diffuser for only about 15 to 20 minutes (depending on the oil), then turn off or unplug. The area in a car is small. You could become nauseous if you do not unplug the diffuser.

Do not smell more than 5 – 6 oils at a time. The reason is the brain may become 'confused' by so many smells.

After smelling the '6th oil', the body may not be able to 'smell' the oil correctly and that may change your perception of the scent.

Do not smell oils straight from the bottle, you should always put a couple of drops of oil on a tissue, paper towel, scent strip and then 'wave' the tissue or scent strip you are using under your nose. Simply take a 'whiff' as the oil goes under your nose.

Have fun and enjoy the world of Aromatherapy!

GLOSSARY

Absolute: a concentrated aromatic extracted from a plant via a multistep process. Extraction involves the use of solvents to produce the first step – a concrete. Alcohol is then used to obtain the final product.

Analgesic: reduces or relieves pain.

Antibacterial: kills or prevents bacterial growth.

Antidepressant: helps relieve depression.

Antifungal: kills or inhibits the growth of fungus

Anti-inflammatory: reduces inflammation

Antimicrobial: inhibits the growth of any variety of microorganisms.

Antiseptic: kills and inhibits the growth of bacteria

Antispasmodic: helps to relieve spasms and cramps.

Antiviral: Kills or weakens viral infections

Aphrodisiac: stimulates sexual arousal and desires

Astringent: reduces secretion and tightens tissues

Carminative: expels gas from the intestinal tract

Carrier or Fixed oil: vegetable-based oil expressed from the nut, seed or flesh of various plants. It is not like the volatile essential oils, as the oil itself does not evaporate into the air.

Cephalic: is pertaining to the head.

Cholagogue: increases bile flow

Cicatrizant: helps the formation of tissue during wound and skin healing.

Decongestant: reduces or relieves congestion

Disinfectant: kills disease-producing microorganisms.

Emmenagogue: deals with menstruation

Essential oil: The aromatic, volatile component produced by plants. It is typically obtained by steam distillation or cold pressing.

Expectorant: helps the lungs and bronchial tubes to thin mucous for easier expulsion.

Febrifuge: helps to reduce fevers

Insecticide: kills insects

Neat: is applied directly without dilution.

Nervine: is a substance that will calm and sooth the nervous system.

Notes: is a method to identify the scents, as they are smelled, along with the various evaporation rates Top, Middle and Base.

Oxidation: The chemical changes resulting when oxygen alters the original chemistry of an organic substance.

Parasitic: kills or controls parasites

Photo sensitive/toxic: is an adverse skin reaction from exposure to sunlight or ultraviolet lights.

Rubefacient: a substance or irritant that will redden the skin

Sedative: promotes drowsiness, or is calming.

Synergy: When you blend two or more essential oils, they can create a substance that is to be more effective as a whole than a sum of the individual components.

Tonic: helps to invigorate the entire body.

Vermifuge: helps to eliminate worms

Vulnerary: helps to heal wounds and sores by applying externally.

About the authors

First, we want to "Thank you" for reading our book.

We are glad you are interested in Aromatherapy, one of the nicest complementary health fields.

Although you may hear it as an Alternative health field we prefer the terminology, COMPLEMENTARY.

Why? We are not here to replace your medical care - rather we are here to help enhance or complement it.

Aromatherapy can make one feel better - physically, mentally and emotionally, and that alone can help you heal yourself from within!

As you search, learn and receive benefits from this ancient form of healing, please feel free to write us with your questions.

Since 1997, we "work" the business. We are the ordering department, the packaging and shipping department, and all the other departments a small business needs. We have fun doing it all!!

We LOVE to give the Personal touch (as many of you know when you have e-mailed us or talked with us on the phone).

We are everyday folks - just like you! We treat you - how we would expect to be treated!

Alan studied aromatherapy through the Australasian College of Herbal Studies. This course has a tough regimen and is one of the Top Three Schools in the USA for Aromatherapy. It is now the "American College of Health Care Sciences".

He will be glad and promptly get you an answer for any question or concern you may have about the use of essential oils.

Penny is the website designer, among many other things. She has been designing web pages for several years now and thoroughly enjoys the creation of the pages. She also helps with advertising and web promotion.

Penny received her certification in Advanced Clinical Aromatherapy in May 2008, which is a very serious course of study in the medical aspects of the use of essential oils for therapeutic aromatherapy.

She enjoys all the therapeutic qualities of the oils as they keep her alert and when done working on the "net", help her to relax. She knows firsthand the benefits of Aromatherapy! She is always learning and studying aromatherapy too.

When Alan and Penny first became interested in Aromatherapy there were very few local (if you call 30 miles away local) places to purchase essential oils (and the oils we did find were of poor quality).

After much thought and many hours and months of research, we decided to start our own Aromatherapy, Essential Oils and Supplies Business.

Again, after much research, we have found suppliers for some of the highest quality oils available today. The oils we sell meet with the highest standards available for quality and purity. Rest assured the oils we sell are of the highest quality oils and are free from adulterations, pesticides and herbicides.

For you, we have done much of the hard work.

After working 20 years in an area hospital (in surgery) and 5 1/2 years at the University of Minnesota Duluth - Facilities Management, and with our Aromatherapy business now consuming more time than Al had to give, he left the University on December 30, 2005 to work on the Aromatherapy business fulltime.

Alan now works many hours each day answering aromatherapy questions by e-mail and by phone. Not to mention all the orders he puts up, printing, restocking and the list continues.

Until recently, Penny worked at a local small animal Veterinary Clinic as an Animal Health Technician and Receptionist. She "retired" from the Veterinary field in June 2004 and has been working the Aromatherapy business full time since then.

Besides our interests in Aromatherapy:
Al loves to read books, golf, riding his recumbent bike, watch movies and fishing.

Penny loves 'surfing' the Internet, her dogs, riding her recumbent bike, watch movies, cook & baking, writing and reading books.

Hope you enjoyed learning a little bit more about us and our aromatherapy business.

Penny and Al Keay

p.s. Our last name is pronounced like the letter "K" - The 'e' is silent.

Made in the USA
Charleston, SC
15 November 2013